YOUR KNOWLEDGE HAS VALUE

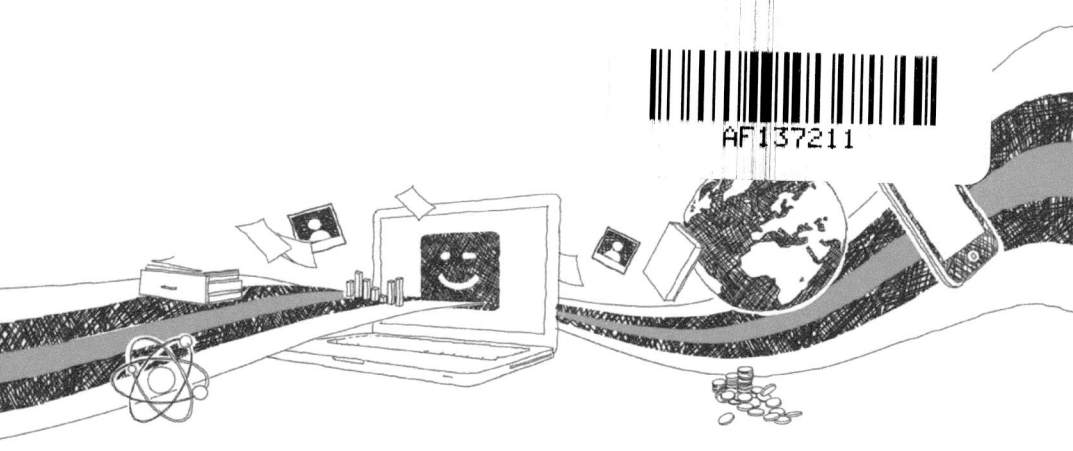

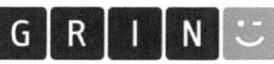

Bibliographic information published by the German National Library:

The German National Library lists this publication in the National Bibliography; detailed bibliographic data are available on the Internet at http://dnb.dnb.de .

Imprint:

Copyright © 2015 GRIN Verlag, Open Publishing GmbH
Print and binding: Books on Demand GmbH, Norderstedt Germany
ISBN: 978-3-668-23761-2

This book at GRIN:

http://www.grin.com/en/e-book/333872/sex-selective-abortion-why-it-should-be-prohibited

Kamalesh Dey

Sex-selective abortion. Why it should be prohibited

GRIN Publishing

GRIN - Your knowledge has value

Since its foundation in 1998, GRIN has specialized in publishing academic texts by students, college teachers and other academics as e-book and printed book. The website www.grin.com is an ideal platform for presenting term papers, final papers, scientific essays, dissertations and specialist books.

Visit us on the internet:

http://www.grin.com/

http://www.facebook.com/grincom

http://www.twitter.com/grin_com

UNIVERSITY OF BEDFORDSHIRE

FACULTY OF HEALTH AND SOCIAL SCIENCES

MSC PUBLIC HEALTH

ETHICAL AND LEGAL ISSUES IN HEALTHCARE
MODULE UNIT CODE: PUB014-6

SUMMATIVE ASSESSMENT

ON

SEX-SELECTIVE ABORTION SHOULD BE PROHIBITED

JANUARY 2014

WORD COUNT: 4339

SEX-SELECTIVE ABORTION SHOULD BE PROHIBITED

INTRODUCTION

The paper will talk about the sex selective abortion and its negative impact on public health. The paper will also critically justify the statement "sex- selective abortion should be prohibited" through different arguments in the perspective of ethical and legal issue of health and social care.

Donaldson and Scally (2009, p.313) stated that "Abortion is defined as the emptying practice of a pregnant uterus up to the twenty four weeks of pregnancy". However, unprompted abortion normally is called miscarriage. Abortion refers to the abolition of a foetus or embryo from uterus just before stage of viability. According to survival statistics, foetus is normally visible within 23 to 24 weeks (Grimes and Stuart, 2010).

Abrejo, Shaikh and Rizvi (2009) defined sex selective abortion is the practice of prenatal discrimination, in which a foetus is aborted just after identifying of its sex. This practice is promoting sex inequality in the society. Moreover, Sex-selective abortion is defined as the termination of pregnancy based on the expected sex of unborn baby. In general, female foetus is the main victim of sex selective abortion in many countries in the world particularly in Southeast Europe, India, Pakistan, People's Republic of China (Goodkind, 1999).

In addition, ethically sex-selective abortion is the illegal and immoral sign of human activities. This action are so harmful for the next generation as high sex ratio imbalance in the community due to only abort of female foetus what ought to be banned under legal law (Cannold, 1994). Though, some countries for instances: United kingdom, Belgium have only limited access of sex selection only for physical status of foetus for instances: physical and mental disability, while Canada, the royal commission of new reproductive technologies claimed that sex selective abortion is an offensive and criminalised under criminal act (Dickens et al., 2005).

Miller (2001) stated that sex selective abortion means abortion of female foetus what is performed mostly in some parts of Asia, particularly in India, China, South Korea, Taiwan, Pakistan and some of Canadian, British and American immigrants.

In United Kingdom, the rate of abortion was increased after legalisation of abortion in 1967. In 2007, the termination of pregnancy rate was about 22%. But, about 60% what was highest abortion rate among young and older women though about 32% among over 40 years' old women (Donaldson and Scally, 2009).

PREVALENCE AND PUBLIC HEALTH IMPACTS OF SEX-SELECTIVE ABORTION

Sex selective abortion is unethical and illegal activities of human being due to advancement of technology. It has great negative impact on public health. Due to abort of female foetus sex ratio is going to high and huge number of men will not have any partner and people will act as broken family and people what would be vicious for the society (Marquis, 2001).

The high prevalence of sex-selective abortion is available in China and India, while sex selective abortion still available some other countries in the world. According to medical research, more than 10 million female foetus have been aborted due to sex selective abortion in the last twenty years in India and around 500 000 girls lost each year due to prenatal selection and sex selective abortion (Ahmad, 2010). In India, according to national census data in 2001, sex ratio was 107.8 males per 100 females what was higher than 1991 when it was 105.8 but some part of India sex ratio was significantly higher. For examples: 126.1 in Punjab and 122.0 in Haryana and 113.9 in Gujarat. Family members balance, son preference theory and cultural and social context in patriarchy society what were the key factors of sex-selective abortion (Arnold, Kishor and Roy, 2002).

In China, sex ratio is quite imbalance due to sex-selective abortion. The average sex ratios were between 103 and 107 among 15 to 19 years age group but much higher among 1-4 years age group children what were 126 in rural areas. In addition, sex ratio was over 130 in six provinces in China and nine provinces had sex ratio more than 160 in rural China what were too high. So, excess numbers of male particularly in all part in China. Consequently, those young people could not have any partners, no wives and they would be isolated from their normal life what could initiate large expansion of sex business and instigate bullying and trafficking. In China and India, recently sex industry has been expanded and recruited huge number of sex workers in china (Zhu, Lu and Hesketh, 2009).

Porter (1994) reported that the rate of abortion about 92 to 96% within the first trimester. Roughly 38 million abortions occurred annually from Latin America, Caribbean, Asia, Africa, and pacific region where more than half abortions performed illegally

Sex-selective abortion tends to imbalance of sex ratio in the society. For the reasons, birth rate of boy will be high; therefore mortality rate would also be higher rather than girl as boy is hereditarily fragile (Kraemer, 2000). Son preference is the main cause of sex selective abortion, though this act leads unpredictable consequences in the society. Basically, East Asia through South Asia to the Middle East and North African countries, son preference is the cultural and traditional norm. Bumgarner (2007) claimed that sons are highly expected rather than girl because of higher earing capacity; continue family line and sign of inheritance, while girls are considered as burden of family as well as in economy because of dowry system and after marriage they traditionally shift to husband's family. An old Indian proverb is known as "Grooming a girl is like watering a neighbour's garden". This spiteful declaration introduced dowry system in the son preference society. For all these points family and society are not willing to get girl. So, they always abort female foetus. Consequently, lots of girls are missing every time from the world what will bring long term impact in the society. Particularly, there are maximum numbers of females disappeared in Indian subcontinent: mostly in Pakistan (about 11%), India (approximately 9.4%), and Bangladesh (almost 8.9% of all disappeared females) due to only sex selective abortion (Hesketh and Xing, 2006).

Lobo and Genuis (2014) reported that trisomy 21 knowing as Down syndrome (DS), learning disability, what is the most common screened condition and prenatal detection in Europe and North America. Lobo and Genuis (2014) also purported that in 2009 about 92% prenatal diagnosed pregnancies were terminated, whereas only 2% due to miscarriage and rest 6% in live birth in United Kingdom. While in North America, 90% pregnancies in Canada and 84 to 91% pregnancy were terminated in United States.

DISCUSSION

Perspective of medical ethics, abortion and sex- selective abortion both performances are quite offensive and awful. In addition, from the viewpoint of ethical and legal issue, abortion means killing someone and what is the central issue of morality (Callahan, 1978)

Particularly, in China and India, are still continuing sex selective abortion as a consequences, sex ratio is much higher what would be irreversible impact on public health and society. Though, sex selective abortion seems to an individual family or parent's interest based on "son preference theory". However, such interest is harm for girl, women as well as whole female society. Consequently, prohibition of sex-selective abortion could only eliminate sex-selective abortion from the son preference society (Zilberberg, 2007).

Vogel (2012) stated that in India, the high imbalance of sex ratio at birth has gradually deteriorated just before the prohibition of sex selective in 2003, while sex of foetus detection testing in 1994. Around three and six million sex selection abortion were completed in India in the year of 2000s, while one and four million in the 1990s and up to two million in 1980s. Similarly, huge number of girls is also missing in China due to only sex selective abortion since 1994. So, both cases only one reason is responsible. So it should be banned under legal law protecting female foetus to life.

Sex selective abortion is unethical and immoral so it is quite impossible for justification through various types of ethics and bio-medical principle. There are several arguments of sex selective abortion what is argued below:

Arguments on Sex-Selective Abortion

There are particular rational arguments based on ethical and legal issues in health care which could be supportive banning sex-selective abortion:

Sex selective abortion is denied and it should be prohibited through the discussing arguments ethically in the view points of various biomedical principles.

According to communitarian, community benefit is more preferable than an individual what might restrict the freedom of individual for long term benefits of the society. Though, selecting sex of foetus is the mother's right, while consideration of the social violence mother's autonomy could be limited. Sex selective abortion should be prohibited for the benefits of whole community in the world. Sex selective abortion is harm for the society due to create imbalance sex ratio and increase the gender discrimination (Beauchamp and Childress, 2001).

Beauchamp and Childress (2001) defined consequentialism is a theory holding such actions what is right or wrong depends on their good and bad consequences. So sex selective action is not supported by consequentialism as such practice leads very bad impact for the society, so it should be prohibited due to reduce the sex imbalance and female inequalities in the society. In addition, virtue ethics and moral theory is the part of consequentialism. Moreover, virtue ethics is the branch of moral philosophy what can evaluate the harm or bad of any actions. So, on both view of point sex abortion is immoral and unethical and sex selective abortion act as social harm so it should be prohibited.

Moreover, sex selective abortion should be restricted in sense of consequentialism. Sex selective abortion still available in some countries where high sex ratio imbalance, particularly in India and china due to strong son preference theory what is highly motivated aborting female foetus enormously. Consequently, high sex ratio is social harm as number of girls is less rather than males. So, high numbers of males will not get any scope having wives or partners in near future, therefore they will have to rely on sex workers for their biological needs what would be shame for whole nation. For that reasons, sex selective abortion is objectionable for raising such hectic problem (McDougall, 2005).

The principle of beneficence always entails positive act, good outcomes and inhibiting bad engagements what is harmful. Alternatively, beneficence eradicates all bad and harmful activities, and stimulates what is moral and well- beneficial. Overall, beneficence is always looking benefits for the user and community (Athar, 2011). Sex selective abortion is not obliged by beneficence as this practice is involved with harmful activities for instance: the killing of foetus, gender discrimination what leads high sex ration imbalance. As a result, next generation will be sufferer in the society. Savulescu (2001) also stated that sex selective abortion leads sex inequality in the society. Principle of beneficence always conflicts with sex inequality and gender discrimination in the society. So, sex selective abortion should be restricted resolving problem from the society, unless gender discrimination would be increased.

The principle of non-maleficence generally involves to safe the person from any kind of harm. The duty of non-maleficence is to rescue the vulnerable person from the predicted harm committed by others intentionally or unintentionally through their activities. So, sex selective abortion is not permissible based on the principle of non-maleficence. According to the duty of non- maleficence, sex selective abortion should be prohibited for saving the female foetus life and giving opportunity for growing up in the womb until born (Gillon, 1994).

Gostin and Gostin (2009) described that "John Stuart Mill's theory of liberty" is occasionally restricted the power of autonomy of an individual once an individual's action is harm for others. Sex-selective abortion obviously harmful action and killing typically female foetus, consequently high sex ratio would be available what could be violent in the society (Jackson, 2000).

Clouser and Gert (1990) stated that morality depends on particular few moral judgements what reply on some parts for instances: moral rules including "don't kill", "don't deceive", "Keep your promise", and "Do your duty"; moral ideas including "preventing death" as well as "releasing pain"; what are the key points of moral judgements. For example: sex selective abortion leads to kill innocent mainly female foetus so based on moral theory this practice should be banned.

Rawls (2009) stated that ethical principle of justice is the real virtue of public organisations where the true thoughts are coming up and judgement based on fairness, while wrong is denied even justice denied also the freedom of person what makes wrong for others. However, mothers have reproduction right making decision to abort but abortion is social harm and killing innocent foetus so according to justice sex selective abortion should be prohibited. Baird (1996) also argued that in view of principle of ethical equality and justice, sex selective abortion is quite unethical. Nevertheless, sex of the foetus is identifiable after 10 weeks pregnancy period. Principles of justice and equality always respect human's life and dignity, though female foetus remains unborn but foetus has right to born in the society. So sex-selective abortion acts as violence in the society. Moreover, Kalfoglou et al. (2013) also claimed that sex-selective abortion is socially unjustified.

Gillon (1994) stated that justice is the fourth prima facie moral principle. Justice is considered making decision with fairness between two competitive claims. In health care ethics, justice is considered generally based on three categories for instances: distributive justice, right based justice (respect for autonomy) and legal justice (morally acceptable law). Legal justice and right based justice both categories of justice would disagree with sex selective abortion. In view point of both categories of justice, sex selective abortion should be prohibited as female foetus has right to live and enjoy her life. Killing female foetus or sex selective abortion both is wrong and immoral. So, sex selective abortion is extremely erroneous due to cruelty killing an innocent foetus what deprived their valuable future and enjoyments of their life in the beautiful world (Steinbock, 2006).

Dickens et al., (2005) stated that sex selective abortion is absolutely injustice. Feminist are also against on sex selective abortion as sex selective abortion is thought to be only appliance and consequences of patriarchy society. However, sex selective abortion is still noticeable in China, Korea and India due to cultural context where son preference theory is extremely adopted. So, high sex ratio imbalance is remaining in those countries. Moreover, the Human Fertilisation and Embryology Authority's public consultation on sperm sorting and pre-implantation genetic diagnosis (PGD) in United Kingdom purported that, 69% people rejected sex selection abortion in 2003 only due to social reasons, while 80% in 1993. Whereas, sex selective abortion is rare among some countries in the world as there is no sex preference for instance: Canada (Dickens et al., 2005).

According to ethical law and public opinion, sex- selective abortion is illegal and immoral activities for the society. So, sex selective abortions should be prohibited for the benefits of human and society (Porter, 1994). Dickens (2002) also stated that sex selective abortion is treated as unethical and illegal performance as killing only female foetus is just like arising gender discrimination and deprived the foetus living in the beautiful world. Moreover, Oomman and Ganatra (2002) indicated that sex selection abortion is unethical. Public health researchers and demographers think that sex selective abortion might decrease the post natal discrimination against girl baby. Sex selective abortion might be substitute of female infanticide what would be harm for female in the society due sex discrimination. So, sex selective abortion should be prohibited.

Sex ratio imbalance is another strong point for illegalised sex-selective abortion. Hvistendahl (2012) reported that sex-selective abortion could be influenced making sex ratio imbalance in the society. Consequently, men do not get any opportunity having partner or wives and no children due to abortion of female foetus in the last decade what would be broken branches condition and disruption of social structure. For protecting such condition as early as possible sex selection abortion should be limited under law (Hudson and Den Boer, 2004). Moreover, Miller (2001) also stated that sex selective abortion leads to make imbalance of sex ratio what act as indicators of the destructions of human right. High sex ratio would make social violence and society would be more likely insecure.

Williams (2012) argued against sex selective abortion as abort female foetus is obviously discrimination against the female foetus what disrupts the principle of sexual equality and it also rejects the equal right of female foetus to life what is quite immoral. So prohibition of sex selective abortion would be only way to resolve this issue.

In sense of religious or divine act, sex selective abortion is highly destructive and sadism motion of human being. claimed that Sex selection of unborn baby is considered as like "playing God". Baby born is a natural process and baby is God gifted from the heaven. According to religious law, Sex selective abortion act is highly objectionable and unacceptable. In addition, in view point of religious view sex selective abortion is offensive as aborting foetus is equivalent killing foetus what is act as impiousness. Moreover, this performance disregards the value of each human being, while collective expression of human being acts as love God. So, sex selective abortion is opposed by all religious organisations (Kalfoglou et al., 2013).

McMahan (2002) argued that sex selective abortion is unjustified and abortion means killing innocent female foetus what is equivalent murdered someone. In addition, sex selective abortion is a sexist and unethical action. Involving with sex selective abortion parents always believe that one sex is much stronger than other, though it depends on particular cultural context. Particularly, in patriarchy society people are normally habituate to choose male foetus rather than female as female are act as burden in son preference society. But, aborting female foetus is unethical as well as social harm for the imbalance sex ratio in society (Strange and Chadwick, 2010).

Vogel (2012) also reported that sex-selective abortion should be prohibited. In India, sex-selective abortion is highly performed so it is known as female feticide. As a result, Government amended punishment law against sex selective abortion under Pre-Conception and Pre-Natal Diagnostic Techniques (Prohibition of Sex Selection) Act 1994. Where, only over 35 age women are permitted accessing prenatal tests with all relevant medical certificates, unless she can be prosecuted. Doctors and parents both will be under sentenced. It may be imprisoned (up to three months) and fined ($320) or both (Ahmad, 2010). Moreover, sex selective abortion is already limited in some countries for instance: South Korea. In South Korea, sex ratio imbalance has reduced significantly due to implementation of prohibition law against sex selective abortion. After that, need much more motivation what can modify their traditional thought (son preference). Prohibition law can reduce the gender discrimination and develop their social and economic status. Education campaign like slogan "love your daughter" would be better for eradicating sex selective abortion from son preference society (Guilmoto, 2007).

Overall, on the basis of all strong arguments sex selective abortion should be prohibited in the society reducing sexual equality and stopping gender discrimination.

However, there are certain negative arguments what might be plausible for legalising sex-selective abortion:

There are only limited following arguments what could only support for legalising sex selective abortion:

According to principle of biomedical ethics "Respect for Autonomy" always prefer freedom of choice and respects individual's right to decide for them what could make better for living (Beauchamp and Childress, 2001). For examples: making right decisions for selecting as personal matter what may be their partner as well as their children. Moreover, if some decisions might be immoral, while there is no right to interrupt as a government unless any harm. Consequently, abortion and sex-selective abortion is obviously choice of mother's (Puri and Nachtigall, 2010).

Moazam (2004) stated that autonomy is the individual right for making their own decision without any kind of influences or coercion what is the key point of bioethics. Respect for autonomy would be great strength of women leading their life well with moral equality without any gender discrimination, race or social class. Moreover, Autonomy could be expanded women's reproductive right what makes flexible generating any decision during pregnancy life. Though, feminists from United States claim that particularly Asian women are depriving from their autonomy for instances: making decision during their pregnancy period, prenatal screening, and sex choice of foetus. However, Asian women's have to give birth boy not girl due to only their cultural and social context what is the evidence of limiting their autonomy, while legal prohibition of sex selective abortion making harm rather than positive consequences (Sherwin,1998).

Moreover, Kalfoglou et al. (2013) stated that women are autonomous and they can abort female foetus as they have right to take decision for performing any activities, while women could be forced mentally to perform sex selective abortion due to social context in their family, husband and communities where women's autonomy would be threatened. In addition, a mother has a right to know the sex of her foetus and know about the physical status of the foetus. According to feminists, women if wish she can abort due to her personal life circumstance. Women can choice as she has right to decide as foetus is inside the womb and womb is the part of mother's body so it her autonomous right, even women have right to selectively abort to reduce the risk of foetal disability or foetal sex (Williams, 2012).

ZILBERBERG (2007) reported that feminists argued on sex selective abortion but actually, almost all of the women are living restricted life where they have no choice, no freedom and no value of autonomy in patriarchy society. Contrariwise, women prefer to abort female foetus only for avoiding see their daughter's life alike them. So they prefer son instead of girl as in patriarchy society son would have better possible life and bring happiness in their family what is the rational choosing son instead of girl. Consequently, for better life women sacrificing their female foetus what is the evidence of moral justice, subsequently there is not necessarily banning then abortion practice. Moreover, adequate enthusiasm through social consultants or offered various incentives to the parents who are willing to abort typically their female foetus. But, it might be plausible to prosecute under abortion law to all involvement of abortion. For examples: health workers, people involved with sex determination test and influential agents. However, women's autonomy might be limited due to only prohibition of sex selective abortion what would be main hindrance of women's reproductive life (Weiss, 1995).

Williams (2012) also claimed that abortion and choosing the sex of foetus is the legal right of women. Feminist philosophers introduced slogan for the women's right " my body, my decision" during pregnancy period making decision is the moral right of all women and no interrupt between decision makings or any execution during pregnancy period. Moreover, Women could decide their own without any coercion, choosing sex of their foetus and no influence of cultural context what will be only the legal moral autonomy. Therefore, Sex selection abortion would be depends on only pregnant mother. Women can also prenatal test identifying the physical status of her foetus and make a plan in their future life. Though, this action is restricted in some countries where sex selective abortion is much more demanding in cultural context. Even, pregnant women could be forced mentally or physically performing sex-selective abortion in particular society where mainly males are highly signified rather than females for instance: India (Baird, 1996).

Strange and Chadwick (2010) claimed that sex selective abortion is preferable to some parents on their social background. Making family balancing, parents could perform sex selective abortion where no risk of psychological harm to anybody as foetus is in non-conscious condition and foetus has no choice only mothers or Parents can decide their preference. So, parents have fundamental right aborting female foetus. Therefore, Sex selective abortion should be legalised making family balance of parents. Moreover, Wertz and Fletcher (1989) claimed that sex choice of foetus would be good chance for parents enhancing the quality of life much better for desire sex of child than undesired. Furthermore, family balance is the strong point as well for son preference. In addition, sex choice is better for mother's life because of only fewer births she has to give, unless she has to wait until their desire child what will be another great problem for growing population. In that sense, sex selective abortion should be legalised for mother's freedom and giving the value of mother's choice. Consequently, sex selective abortion might be justified for prenatal diagnosis for identifying and prevention of serious genetic disease. So, banning sex selective abortion would be threatened for reproductive freedom of women where their genetic knowledge could be abused (Nelson, 2000).

Finally, sex selective abortion should not ban especially perspective of women's autonomy unless women's reproductive right would be endangered.

CONCLUSION

Prohibition of Sex selective abortion is argued based on ethical and legal issue, whereas prohibition of sex selective abortion is justified through all biomedical principles except principle of Autonomy. As, Autonomy only argued against prohibition law of sex selective abortion, because of women have reproductive freedom and they have right to abort and choosing sex of foetus. However, prohibition law is justified through all biomedical principle and mostly sex selective abortion is scrutinised as an unethical, immoral and illegal practice due to its negative consequences in many countries in the world for instances: India, China, and South Korea. High sex ratio is the major problem promoting gender inequality in those areas. So, strictly adaptation of prohibition law could be feasible solution of raised problem. For example: prohibition of sex selective abortion law is activated in south Korea, consequently sex ratio is reducing gradually as positive outcome. Therefore, sex selective abortion should be prohibited minimising sex inequalities, gender discrimination and establish the right of the female innocent foetus to life in the beautiful world.

REFERENCES

Abrejo, F.G., Shaikh, B.T. and Rizvi, N. (2009) "And they kill me, only because I am a girl'...a review of sex-selective abortions in south Asia', European Journal of Contraception and Reproductive Health Care, 14 (1), pp.10-16 [online]. Available at: http://0-eds.b.ebscohost.com.brum.beds.ac.uk/eds/pdfviewer/pdfviewer?sid=084ad7f4-388d-4b01-946d-432476a332f4%40sessionmgr114&vid=1&hid=111 (Accessed: 20 December 2014).

Ahmad, N. (2010) 'Female feticide in India', Issues in Law and Medicine, 26 (1), pp.13-29 [online]. Available at: http://0-eds.b.ebscohost.com.brum.beds.ac.uk/eds/pdfviewer/pdfviewer?sid=c692aee4-8c52-4ede-9cdc-9b87a11a753b%40sessionmgr111&vid=1&hid=111 (Accessed: 15 January 2015).

Arnold, F., Kishor, S. and Roy, T. (2002) 'Sex-Selective abortions in India', Population and Development Review, 28 (4), pp.759-785 [online]. Available at: http://onlinelibrary.wiley.com/doi/10.1111/j.1728-4457.2002.00759.x/pdf (Accessed: 15 January 2015).

Athar, S. (2011) 'Principles of biomedical ethics', The Journal of IMA, 43 (3), pp.138 [online]. Available at: http://www.ncbi.nlm.nih.gov/pmc/articles/PMC3516124/pdf/jima-43-3-8476.pdf (Accessed: 16 January 2015).

Baird, P.A. (1996) 'Ethical issues of fertility and reproduction', Annual Review of Medicine, 47 pp.107-116 [online]. Available at: http://0-eds.b.ebscohost.com.brum.beds.ac.uk/eds/pdfviewer/pdfviewer?sid=d0c4ff3c-fbea-40b0-a461-370f374bdbe2%40sessionmgr114&vid=1&hid=111 (Accessed: 5 January 2015).

Beauchamp, T.L. and Childress, J.F. (2001) Principles of biomedical ethics. Fifth edn. New York: Oxford university press.

Bumgarner, A. (2007) 'Right to choose: Sex selection in the international context, A', Duke J.Gender L.and Pol'y, 14 pp.1289 [online]. Available at: http://scholarship.law.duke.edu/cgi/viewcontent.cgi?article=1139&context=djglp&sei-redir=1&referer=http%3A%2F%2Fscholar.google.co.uk%2Fscholar%3Fhl%3Den%26q%3DA%2Bright%2Bto%2Bchoose%253F%2BSex%2Bselection%2Bin%2Bthe%2Binternational%2Bcontext%26btnG%3D%26as_sdt%3D1%252C5%26as_sdtp%3D#search=%22right%20choose%3F%20Sex%20selection%20international%20context%22 (Accessed: 20 January 2015).

Callahan, D. (1978) 'Abortion and medical ethics', The Annals of the American Academy of Political and Social Science, 437 (1), pp.116-127[online]. Available at: http://www.jstor.org/stable/pdfplus/1042498.pdf (Accessed: 20 January 2015).

Cannold, L. (1994) 'Consequences for patients of health care professionals' conscientious actions: The ban on abortions in South Australia', Journal of Medical Ethics, 20 (2), pp.80-86 [online]. Available at: http://0-www.jstor.org.brum.beds.ac.uk/stable/27717400 (Accessed: 10 January 2015).

Clouser, K.D. and Gert, B. (1990) 'A critique of principlism', *The Journal of Medicine and Philosophy,* 15 (2), pp.219-236 [online]. Available at: http://jmp.oxfordjournals.org/content/15/2/219.full.pdf (Accessed: 5 January 2015) .

Dickens, B.M. (2002) 'Can sex selection be ethically tolerated?', Journal of Medical Ethics, 28 (6), pp.335-336.

Dickens, B.M. (2002) 'Can sex selection be ethically tolerated?', *Journal of Medical Ethics,* 28 (6), pp.335-336 [online]. Available at: http://jme.bmj.com/content/28/6/335.full.pdf+html (Accessed: 10 January 2015)

Dickens, B.M., Serour, G.I., Cook, R.J. and Qiu, R.-. (2005) 'Sex selection: Treating different cases differently', *International Journal of Gynecology and Obstetrics,* 90 (2), pp.171-177 [online]. Available at: http://0-www.sciencedirect.com.brum.beds.ac.uk/science/article/pii/S0020729205002912 (Accessed: 4 January 2015).

Donaldson, L.J. and Scally, G. (2009) Donaldsons' essential public health. Third edn. United Kingdom: Radcliffe Publishing.

Gillon, R. (1994) 'Medical ethics: Four principles plus attention to scope', *BMJ (Clinical Research Ed.),* 309 (6948), pp.184-188 [online]. Available at: http://www.ncbi.nlm.nih.gov/pmc/articles/PMC2540719/pdf/bmj00449-0050.pdf (Accessed: 10 January 2015).

Goodkind, D. (1999) 'Should prenatal sex selection be restricted? ethical questions and their implications for research and policy', Population Studies, 53 (1), pp.49-61[online]. Available at: http://www.jstor.org/stable/2584811?seq=1#page_scan_tab_contents (Accessed: 20 December 2014).

Gostin, L.O.(.1.). and Gostin, K.G.(.2.). (2009) 'A broader liberty: J.S. mill, paternalism and the public's health', *Public Health,* 123 (3), pp.214-221.

Grimes, D.A. and Stuart, G. (2010) 'Abortion jabberwocky: The need for better terminology', Contraception, 81 (2), pp.93-96.

Guilmoto, C. (2007) 'Sex-ratio imbalance in Asia: Trends, consequences and policy responses', *Paris: LPED/IRD,[online].* Available at: http://www.unfpa.org/sites/default/files/resource-pdf/regional_analysis.pdf (Accessed: 20 January 2015).

Hesketh, T. and Xing, Z.W. (2006) 'Abnormal sex ratios in human populations: Causes and consequences', *Proceedings of the National Academy of Sciences of the United States of America,* 103 (36), pp.13271-13275 [online]. Available at: http://0-www.jstor.org.brum.beds.ac.uk/stable/30050776 (Accessed: 20 January 2015).

Hudson, V.M. and Den Boer, A. (2004) *Bare branches: The security implications of Asia's surplus male population.* Cambridge, MA, USA: MIT Press.

Hvistendahl, M. (2012) *Unnatural selection: Choosing boys over girls, and the consequences of a world full of men.* United States: Public Affairs.

Jackson, E. (2000) 'Abortion, autonomy and prenatal diagnosis', *Social & Legal Studies,* 9 (4), pp.467-494 [online]. Available at: http://sls.sagepub.com/content/9/4/467.full.pdf+html (Accessed: 10 January 2015).

Kalfoglou, A.L., Kammersell, M., Philpott, S. and Dahl, E. (2013) 'Ethical arguments for and against sperm sorting for non-medical sex selection: A review ', *Reproductive Biomedicine Online,* 26 (3), pp.231-239 [online.] Available at: http://0-www.sciencedirect.com.brum.beds.ac.uk/science/article/pii/S147264831200692X (Accessed: 9 January 2015) .

Kraemer, S. (2000) 'The fragile male', *BMJ (Clinical Research Ed.),* 321 (7276), pp.1609-1612.

Lobo, R. and Genuis, G. (2014) 'Socially repugnant or the standard of care: Is there a distinction between sex-selective and ability-selective abortion?', *Canadian Family Physician Médecin De Famille Canadien,* 60 (3), pp.212-216 [online]. Available at: http://0-eds.b.ebscohost.com.brum.beds.ac.uk/eds/pdfviewer/pdfviewer?sid=f46bc93b-0a07-4649-8a18-662dac5d3ee6%40sessionmgr113&vid=1&hid=111 (Accessed: 21 January 2015).

Marquis, D. (2001) 'Deprivations, futures and the wrongness of killing ', *Journal of Medical Ethics,* 27 (6), pp.363-369.

McDougall, R. (2005) 'Acting parentally: An argument against sex selection', *Journal of Medical Ethics,* 31 (10), pp.601-605 [online]. Available at: http://www.jstor.org/stable/pdfplus/27719494.pdf (Accessed; 22 January 2015).

McMahan, J. (2002) *the ethics of killing: Problems at the margins of life.* New York: Oxford University Press.

Miller, B.D. (2001) 'Female-selective abortion in Asia: Patterns, policies, and debates', American Anthropologist, 103 (4), pp.1083 [online]. Available at: http://0-eds.b.ebscohost.com.brum.beds.ac.uk/eds/command/detail?sid=6556661b-41d5-4504-a885-744571ca52c5%40sessionmgr115&vid=1&hid=111 (Accessed: 15 January 2015).

Moazam, F. (2004) 'Feminist discourse on sex screening and selective abortion of female foetuses', *Bioethics,* 18 (3), pp.205-220 [online]. Available at: http://onlinelibrary.wiley.com/doi/10.1111/j.1467-8519.2004.00390.x/pdf (Accessed: 20 January 2015).

Nelson, J.L. (2000) 'Reproductive ethics and the family', *New Zealand Bioethics Journal,* 1 (1), pp.4-10.

Oomman, N. and Ganatra, B.R. (2002) 'Sex selection: The systematic elimination of girls', *Reproductive Health Matters,* 10 (19), pp.184-188 [online]. Available at: http://ac.els-cdn.com/S0968808002000290/1-s2.0-S0968808002000290-main.pdf?_tid=8406e922-a1c8-11e4-8f8a00000aacb360&acdnat=1421884510_ad3f2b0ef26907d758081e06ab470c8c (Accessed: 3 January 2015.)

Porter, E. (1994) 'Abortion ethics: Rights and responsibilities', *Hypatia,* 9 (3), pp.66-87[online]. Available at: http://0-www.jstor.org.brum.beds.ac.uk/stable/3810189 (20 January 2015).

Puri, S. and Nachtigall, R.D. (2010) 'the ethics of sex selection: A comparison of the attitudes and experiences of primary care physicians and physician providers of clinical sex selection services', *Fertility and Sterility,* 93 (7), pp.2107-2114.

Rawls, J. (2009) *A theory of justice.* Revised edn. United States of America: Harvard university press.

Savulescu, J. (2001) 'Procreative beneficence: Why we should select the best children', *Bioethics,* 15 (5-6), pp.413-426 [online]. Available at: http://onlinelibrary.wiley.com/doi/10.1111/1467-8519.00251/pdf (Accessed: 10 January 2015).

Sherwin, S. (1998) *the politics of women's health: Exploring agency and autonomy.* United States of America: Temple University Press.

Steinbock, B. (2006) 'The morality of killing human embryos', *Journal of Law, Medicine and Ethics,* 34 (1), pp.26 [online]. Available at: http://0-eds.b.ebscohost.com.brum.beds.ac.uk/eds/pdfviewer/pdfviewer?sid=fd48b29a-72ef-4106-8ccf-5212746bbe14%40sessionmgr111&vid=2&hid=111 (Accessed: 6 January 2015).

Strange, H. and Chadwick, R. (2010) 'The ethics of nonmedical sex selection', *Health Care Analysis,* 18 (3), pp.252-266 [online]. Available at: http://0-eds.b.ebscohost.com.brum.beds.ac.uk/eds/pdfviewer/pdfviewer?sid=414a4c77-3b70-4d82-a53a-f05b2baafd89%40sessionmgr111&vid=1&hid=111 (Accessed: 20 January 2015) .

Vogel, L. (2012) 'Sex-selective abortions: No simple solution': *Canadian Medical Association Journal = Journal De l'Association Medicale Canadienne,* 184 (3), pp.286-288.

Weiss, G. (1995) 'Sex-Selective abortion: A relational approach', *Hypatia,* 10 (1), pp.202-217 [online]. Available at: http://www.jstor.org/stable/pdfplus/3810465.pdf (Accessed: 20 January 2015)

Wertz, D.C. and Fletcher, J.C. (1989) 'Fatal knowledge? prenatal diagnosis and sex selection', *Hastings Center Report,* 19 (3), pp.21-27 [online]. Available at: http://www.jstor.org/stable/pdfplus/3562739.pdf (Accessed: 201 January 2015).

Williams, J. (2012) 'Sex-selective abortion: A matter of choice', *Law and Philosophy,* 31 (2), pp.125-159 [online]. Available at: http://0-eds.b.ebscohost.com.brum.beds.ac.uk/eds/pdfviewer/pdfviewer?sid=f4e653e8-20df-451b-8e81-77ee4324e9a6%40sessionmgr112&vid=1&hid=111(Accessed: 16 January 2015).

Zhu, W.X., Lu, L. and Hesketh, T. (2009) 'China's excess males, sex selective abortion, and one child policy: Analysis of data from 2005 national inter-census survey', *BMJ (Clinical Research Ed.),* 338 pp.b1211 [online]. Available at: http://www.bmj.com/content/338/bmj.b1211(Accessed: 20 January 2015)

Zilberberg, J. (2007) 'Sex selection and restricting abortion and sex determination', *Bioethics,* 21 (9), pp.517-519.

YOUR KNOWLEDGE HAS VALUE

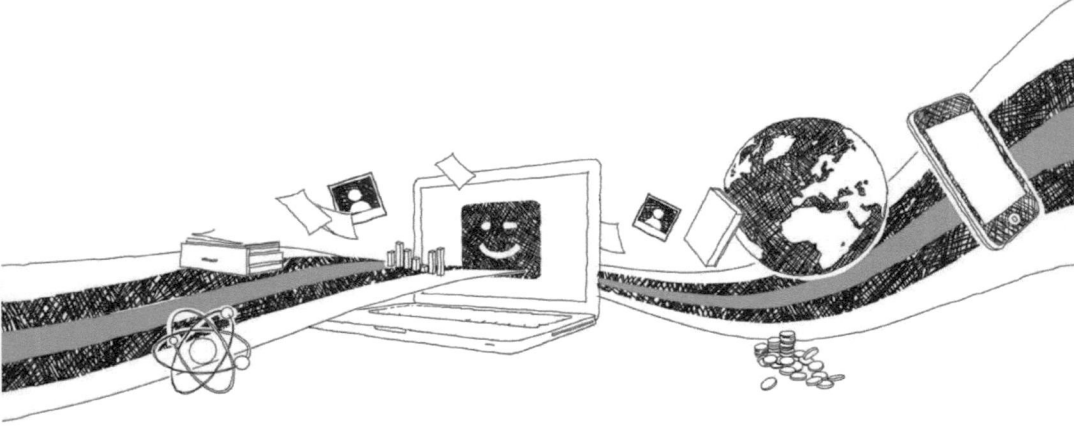

- We will publish your bachelor's and master's thesis, essays and papers

- Your own eBook and book - sold worldwide in all relevant shops

- Earn money with each sale

Upload your text at www.GRIN.com and publish for free

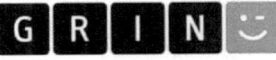